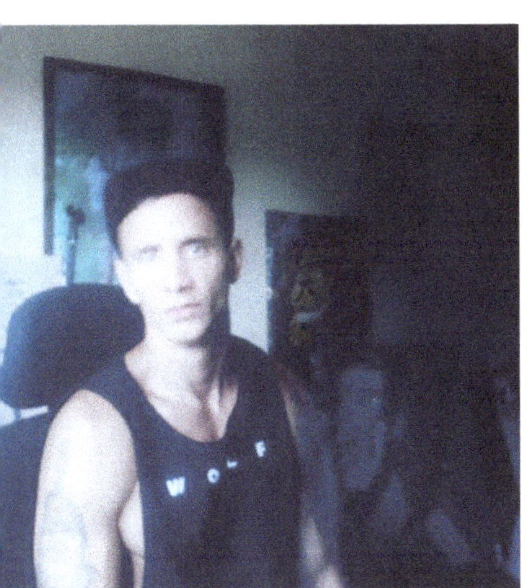

THE MIND MATTERS

ProcsArt

IMPRESSIONIST ART

Keeping your mind occupied, busy and methodical. Taking rest breaks, nutrition, 5 a day and staying hydrated plays a huge part in how we think, speak and act.

Justin Johnson (author/artist)

Mental Health & Wellbeing/ First edition!

The Mind Matters

The Mind Matters

#Mental Health advocate

#Mental Health Ambassador

We all have Mental Health &
Well-being,

Sleep & Nutrition plays a huge part in how we feel and act, we will act accordingly in how we sleep and control our diet. Money worry's, debt worry's, relationships worry's, family disputes etc..

Are you a sufferer of Mental Health Illness?

Would you ask for help?

Everyone at some stage of their life weather that be a bereavement, broken heart, and addiction, lifelong illness, separation from marriage, miscarriage. Your children with disability. Fatal injury at work or even doing the sport or hobbies you enjoy, but now due to injury you cannot fulfil your compassion.

Now is the time to start to think how can we rebuild our thinking pattern around the adaptations of our injury or loss?

Time & Forbearance is the cure for many things, but we need another focus in life to keep us occupied.

I want you to plan, a future ‘a goal’ have a vision! Because success is triumphant. You need some get up and go, or you won’t get up!

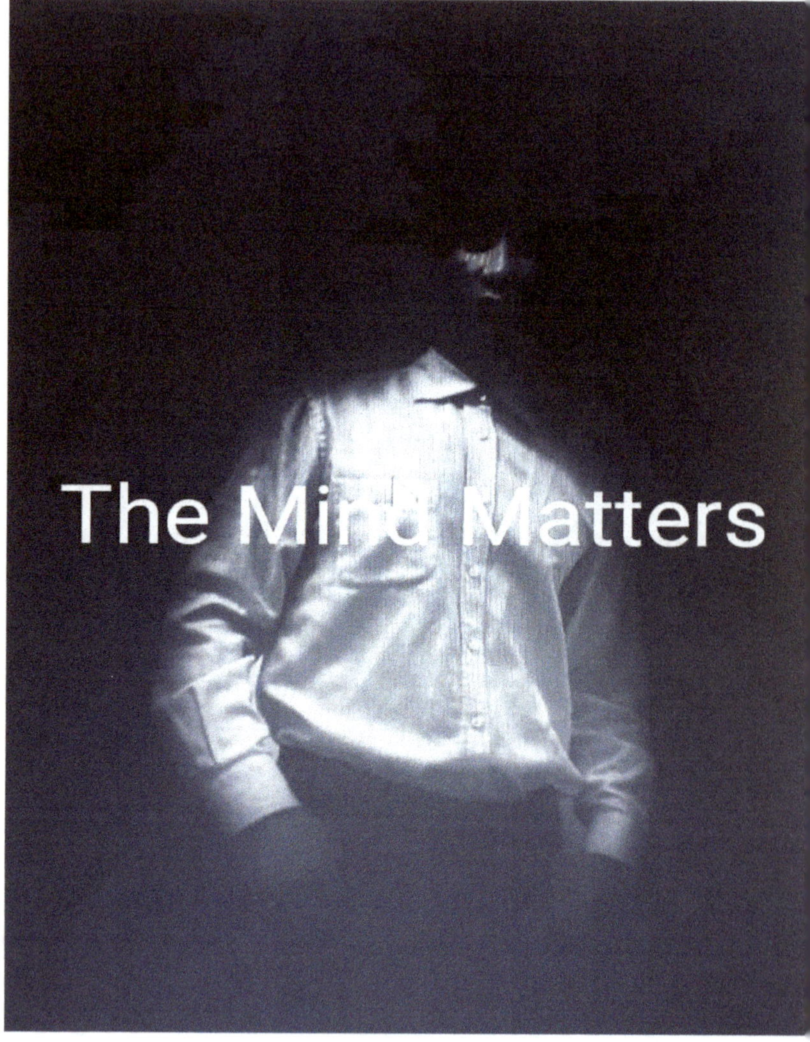

Writer/Author/J.Johnson

Author/Writer J.Johnson (copywrited). Central Committee Representive for Social Science & Arts Faculty @OpenUniversity

Finished 16/08/2022

An Academic Integrity of Arts and humanity, Ungraduated Mature Student

The Mind Matter's blueprint:

1. Anxiety
2. Depression
3. Captivating
4. Striking
5. Empathy
6. Helpful
7. Compassion
8. Motivational
9. Desirable
10. Mental Health & Wellbeing
11. Vitality
12. Flourishing
13. Nourishing

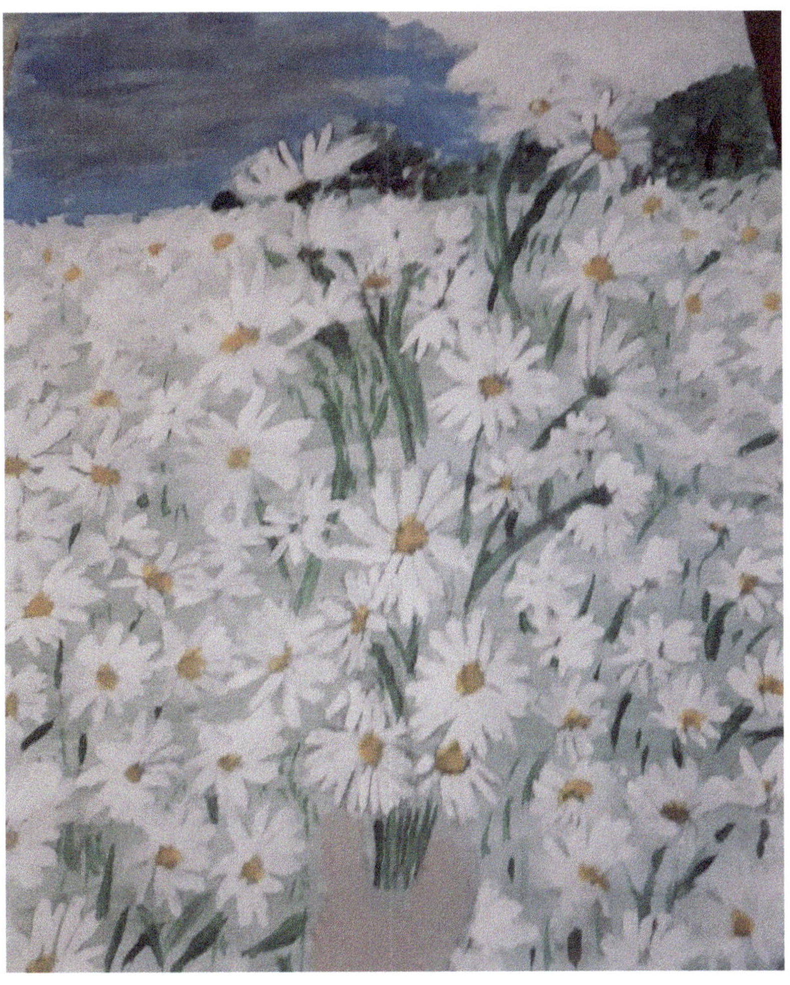

Contemporary Impressionist Art by ProcsArt, Daffodil scenery

I am a firm believer we need to stay methodical to live a balanced lifestyle, we need to adhere to certain situations whether that be through, relationships, business, home life, hobbies, or interests.

Three simple rules of life

1) If you don’t go after what you want, you’ll never get it.
2) If you don’t ask for what you want out of life the answer is always no.
3) If you don’t take a step forward, you always be standing in the same place

The name given; Justin is a masculine given name of, the Latin origin. It is the anglicized form of the Latin given name Justinus, a derivative of Justus, meaning 'Just' 'Fair', or 'righteous'. Justinus was the name borne by various early saints, notably a 2nd-Century Christian' apologist and a boy martyr of the 3rd century, Boy Martyr sums up my life proficiency.

'The Theophilus of Christianity'

As I live the life with the Big Black Dog on my shoulder, but as I carry it in turn, and with faith & hope

With the introduction at thought I want to draft a good Chemical-balance which will help you feel triumphant and draft up some bad examples!

I am a sufferer of depression and anxiety so I will give some examples of the situations I had struggled with.

There is no exterior motive to why I want to discover this book, no other than my compassion for humanity!

(Supporting our People)

To a better way of thinking Action Plan.

Writer/Author/J.Johnson

Do not be afraid to talk about or ask for help with mental health or anxiety, do not feel like you are exacerbating some sort of pestilence,

Feeling emotional or suffering mental health because it is not a weakness, it is not a label and people should not judge you if you need support!

Ask your GP for help?

If you feel that your GP is not helping you with your situation enough, ask for further help with the NHS. Speak about the different avenues you can go about getting the right support!

Judgmental people can run a further risk of you deterioration, so having those circles of friends could b the route to the problem, surround yourself with positiv people who will only support you, the ones that want t see you excel at life! Positiveness has all th fundamentals to happiness!

Surround yourself with people you want to drink your cup of tea with!

A chemical imbalance

How can you acknowledge an impairment to your mental health?

The sense of negativity, the thought of failure, is the biggest sense of fear. We all search for accomplishments, the triumphant feeling factor of winning.

I want to keep the focus on what makes us feel not accepting our thoughts, feeling disorientated. Do you wake up in the morning not knowing how to start your day? If the answer is a, no?

That is the start of a negative downward spiral, staying methodical in practice is a highly motivational perspective! I want to stress the fact that sleep is incredibly important as lack of sleep will make you fatigued, sometimes miserable and stressed. Your thinking mechanism becomes delayed or delusional, putting your shoes on forgetting your tie. Sending a formal email but forgetting the date or the addressee, even the title/headline of the email! You have sent a formal email now with no headline to the main body of information, which could mean the message becoming irrelevant or being missed! Everyday composure is the importance of acceptance, the acceptance of one's self-esteem, for accomplishments! Plenty of sufficient sleep, having a vision, striving ambition, and not fearing failure or rejection.

The Common Cause of depression?

A general cause of depression can be stress which tends to be the worry of money, debts, relationships, the fear of homelessness or bereavement of loss of family which sometimes can lead to feeling suicidal and some may like to suggest parental alienation is a massive conductor of distress leading to deep depression can also lead to feeling very suicidal.

How to signal depression coming into depression or the thought of depression?

Not acknowledging taste of foods, loss of smell, such as perfumes the sweet smell of autumn Cut grass and fallen Leaf's, some of the main essentials to the sweet ascetics of life, these are the living empathetic organics to nature's escapism! Have you ever been listening to your favourite music track, then to realize you have not even acknowledged the words, the musical instruments played during the time of deep depression at thought instead, something your mind will not accept is to engage with happiness rather than focus on what is caused you the provocation to a distress.

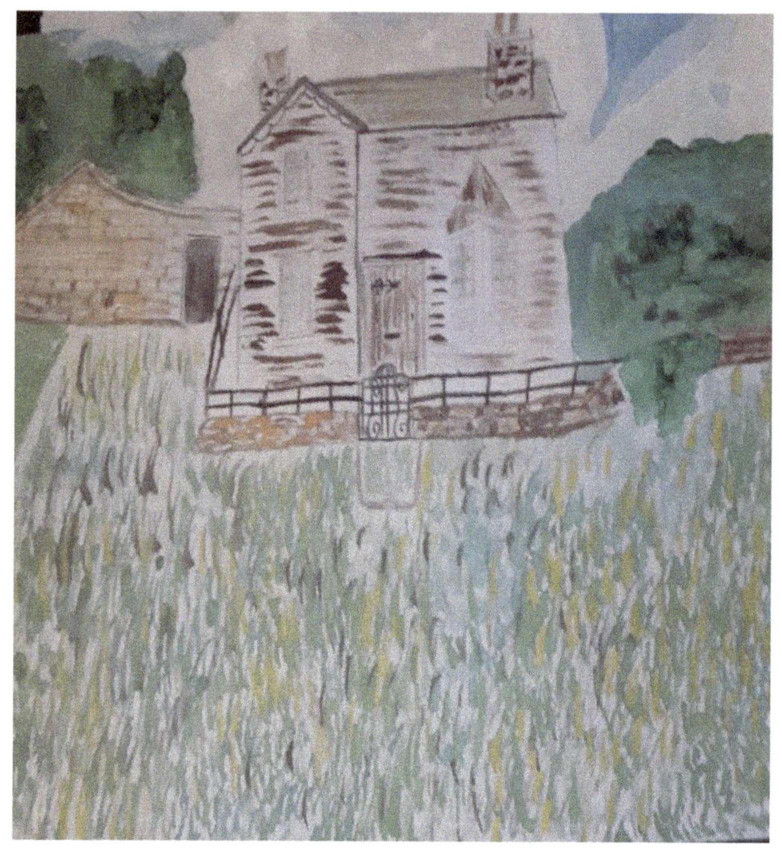

Contemporary Impressionist landscape building art Via ProcsArt

Understanding yourself?

Introvert or Extrovert?

Understanding yourself will help you acknowledge people and whom you like to be surrounded by,

For instance, are you an introvert or extrovert?

An extrovert is an extremely outgoing and full of confidence type of person

Introvert is a shy reticent person, more than likely most people who suffer from not being able to adapt friendships or relationships so easily as they tend to lack confidence!

This does not mean to say an extrovert will not suffer anxiety and depression at some stage of their lives. But being outgoing and confident will help them strive in many situations and get out of boredom a lot easier!

At times I would say I am a bit of both, but formally as a youth I was very much an introvert, my younger years and growing into an adult my athleticism has kept me engaged with humanity.

I am now retired from athleticism due to deteriorating and old age! Being an introvert can have many struggles with finding a relationship or friendship suddenly throughout our life finding a compatible relationship which you tenaciously tend to not be wanting to let go off as the hope of finding another likeminded person can be a rarity, both shy people, how do you go about asking the other to a date to your local coffee shop or a fancy restaurant? These are some of the main struggles an introvert will face and come across. Which makes us very observant for other things in life, critical thinkers, readers, writers. What one lacks within introvert or extrovert the other gains other keys skills the other does not necessarily have much strength with. An extrovert tends to be full of confidence and talk's a good talk but fundamentally not so great with the key skills an introvert shy person has. From a Males perspective to date a woman, the female usually would prefer her man to be full of confidence, I mean who would not? Say you have been single for some years, all you need is a comforter due to loneliness, so someone who is outspoken confident to ask you out on a date and full of conversation will always outgive an introvert

Example of what might happen if an Introvert and Extrovert get together?

When an extrovert can make an Introvert left feeling perturbed or inadequate, the extrovert's confidence, let us say the extrovert is the male, the dominant alfa male type, full of wit and charm, Hes got the swag Hes got the charm, and he has the walk, he goes up to the introvert female, ‘alryt luv your looking ravishing today beautiful, with such elegance, ermm fancy a date, our local café for coffee, tea, we could get to know one another a bit better, since everyone outside here can see what’s going on here,, if not take my number? Mm ok she goes nervously, she reaches for her pocket nervously to get her phone, ok go on then she goes, ohh great lovely job fire away he goes, kk 07865433211 she says. Nice thanks darling i will give you a call and arrange this coffee in the week luv, yeah’ is that alryt? Yes, she says impishly knowing that she gave him the wrong number. This is a usual emotion on how an introvert would act in a situation such as this. I am not sure whether you are the same, if you are an introvert yourself, majority of us now days use the social media or dating sites to communicate when we get to the point of loneliness, it is a fantastic way of meeting somebody that matches your preferences, such as they usually have a bio, saying if they drink, take narcotics, their hobbies, and interests. As an introvert I am not a social person. Many of us will have to take safety precautions by previous experiences or catfishes, many of people will use false identity with a photoshopped profile picture. Or their personality is not as equipped as their bio reads. For many of you it may be worth checking their government name and then comparing the evidence given to see if it matches up with Claire's law. Claires Law is provided by a Police report which keeps track of the personal behaviour report, such as crimes, theft, burglary, rape, violence etc..

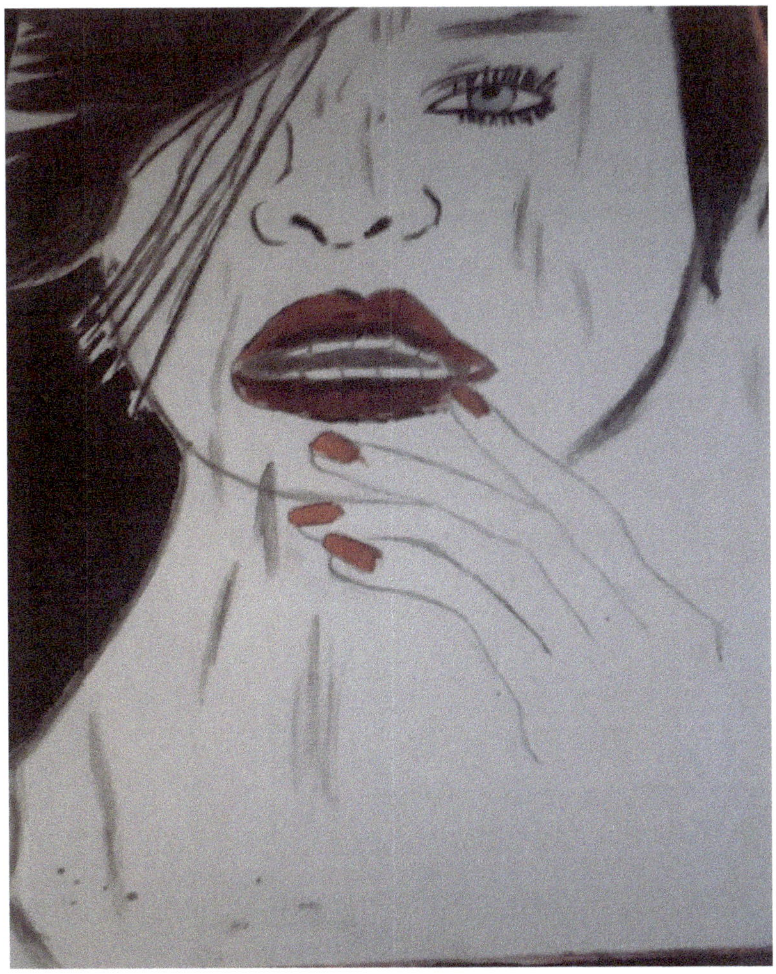

<u>Contemporary Impressionist Art, The pure elegance of feminism via ProcsArt Change!</u>

Change can also be another key focus on a change in mood circumstances, a change of roll at work for instances, your mind becomes with shock or worry, your mind is used like a computer mechanism working methodical in practice, imagine buying new software for your laptop or desktop? Precisely it takes time to learn new applications and sometimes takes further learning or computer courses on key functional skills to be able to fully access its program. Not knowing your work routine, the day that you attend your workplace can leave you feeling be-twixt, thoughts on anxiety or depression of not knowing what your day has planned out by your boss's new Rota.

Change of circumstances in or out of a Relationship and evidence of both concepts

Let us begin with understanding how our mind works when it becomes attracted to the opposite sex, or same sex for some of us! This may not be the same feeling in general for all of us as some may have more offers for dating than others. Which could be due to hunger for lust and compassion with several opportunities. Here I am not trying to become stereotypical as all humanity is capable of anything and everything if the leash is taken off or circumstances to their lifestyle can alter. Now our focus is the question (Depression & Anxiety), Anxiety can accrue in many strange ways such as your next date, say you have been out of practice on dating for years?

You meet a local girl or a girl near or far perhaps at a fair location between the two of you? On a dating site you trade messages back and forth, you find you both have had a bad previous relationship with many things in common. This gives you the sense that it will become amicable between you providing you both attracted to one another on the day, as either of you could be a troll come date night to one that does not meet the other's eye. We both know that our profile pictures would be our best presentable photogenic perception of ourselves. So, on the night before the date it will not become unusual for most of us to start feeling anxious about meeting up with one another.

Both hoping that they will accept and approve of each other's perception of qualities, dress sense, personality and looks. Another sense of comparability could come as one is more competent at dating than the other, which will leave negativity between them. The competent one could be for instance more eager than the other, the dinner date went overwhelmingly well, the conversation got flowing as the night drew near, time comes as they must part ways at the station of arrival meeting point, they say their goodbyes, but the male competent one goes to kiss her goodbye which is significantly the turning point to the shy one's anxiety from reaching its turning point. The next protocol from the male's perspective is to organize another date with her as he found her attractive, but his competence puts off the girl's ideas of completely as confidence can make the lady feel undesirable! As in her mind her thoughts exactly, is he doing the same thing to many girls dating and kissing on first date? ***The dominance of man can fear the confidence of woman!*** This can happen in so many situations with male and female, the male being like the wild boar overconfident and not patient or understanding enough to take things step by step. **Time and forbearance are the best purity to most commodities within the brain's thinking and repairing mechanism, leaving time is of essence to let the male and female grow or nature to one another's feelings! (Time and Forbearance) is also a cure for anxiety and depression, this can lead to how we can deal with situations trying to learn to live with it and learn to deal with something therapeutic which helps the mind adhere to concentration!** Preparation for academic studies, having interest or hobbies is the most relevant materials to combine a focus, this should help calm the feeling of anxiousness or a distress from stress, whilst your mind is occupied with relevance as above, it then adheres to control! I am not saying in down time or after finishing for the day that anxiety will not creep up again but possibly and eventually you may manage your situation of anxiety or depression more sufficiently

The interior Motives of Depression and Anxiety?

Some of this evidence and principles are opinionated facts from my thoughts of different situations we may face in our day-to-day lives. I am hoping with our write up of evidence we can relate with what might be the cause of our depression and what may be the cause of anxiety, I feel like depression can come in a form of deep thought of something we fear or have lost, and anxiety is something that we feel which can make us go into a panic station.

I feel like anxiety may be something for instance that we await to happen, let me give an easy simple prime example, such as we are waiting for the phone alarm to go off for when we finish for work, to then go the theatre with a friend or girlfriend. Watching the clock's hands move around the dial, looking at the phone, alarm still not made a sound, seconds, minutes, hours! This feeling is anxiety can make your bladder become irritable, irritable even to the moment your alarm goes off and you are finally home preparing to get changed from work into your night best wear for your evening at the theatre! Your anxiety will not leave you until you arrive at the Theatres destination simply because what is on at the Theatre has a time schedule to work too, for the publication to be screened by set time, Same as catching a flight, you have a time frame, to catch a flight to go abroad with family. If there is a road closed along the way to the airport and you find that you did not plan your route beforehand you could become late for arrival of departure, this again is another example of great anxiety!

Anxiety and Depression *are both very complexed words remarkably similar in comparison as one can tend to lead to the other, with a mix up of a few of anxiety's failures examples will lead to depression. Depression as we know comes as a form of failure, so imagine planning both theatre and trip abroad and both go wrong as suggested above, missing the time slots provided, which then can become costly, let us say a month's wages or more spent for both, I mean how much would it take for us to work and save a month's wages, a year as a guesstimate, providing we have general household to keep such as bills etc. Some of us can shrug of failure better than others, weather that be pure temperament of the individual or a social class! Money is a massive influence on us all to find happiness or plain escapism from reality, such stress away from home life or work. Our everyday duties.*

Can money buy Anxiety or depression deprivation?

The facts are yes money can buy Anxiety and Depression in many forms, not every single aspect but most certainly quit a few, Money can provide if you have so much of it not having to work for someone else, so this instance having staff to run your business, so that you can plan to get away with ever you feel it is necessary. Your bills will be covered by your finances. You could plan to stay at a hotel the night before your flight abroad to make sure you cover your trip to board the flight on time. I do not believe money can fully justify all aspects of anxiety and depression but certainly give you a wider option to deal with things better such as depression, as a loss of family member would always become a devastation to anyone, but the fact you can find escapism with money which might help the mind escape for a short while, enough to help your mind repair and how to deal with recovery easier!

I do not want everyone to believe that money is everything, as we know we cannot take money with us when we die. But it can help life chances with either anxiety or depression becoming manageable or easier if dealt with appropriately! Some people can fall into depression or have anxiety and cannot cope, their coping mechanism is structured with hurt, so they may sin to take their pain away, such as alcoholism or narcotics. This chemical imbalance will lead to further complications of feeling more anxiousness and deeper depression, to nausea, insomnia, psychosis, with nausea and insomnia together making you feel suicidal or imaginary to what might be there with you but not actually in the room, nausea making you feel like or vomiting, running the risk of losing appetite and losing weight or even Sicking up blood. Insomnia is loss of sleep, which is caused by cholesteryl, too much sugar in alcohol, or even affective A class narcotics which act to an additive effect to speed up and enjoy the night life. Having Psychosis can make you a danger to yourself and society, it is a severe mental disorder in which the thoughts and emotions are so impaired that your contact becomes lost with eternal life.

Stress is related to the cause of anxiety and depression, the thought of worry and change.

A change in so many circumstances such as job preferences for instance. A new job title or job position can mean a few things, learning to work a new routine or program! Working in a different area of the workplace means you will have to make new friends' This thought of worrying about the next day at work can become overwhelming, to learn a new routine and make new friends. You and I both know it will take time to adapt to change, will you have a good relationship with the unfamiliar staff in your new working department?

Let us draft some more examples to compare evidence, hoping you can relate to at least some of these topics spoken about.

Let us suggest social divisions within the household as when we were children growing up with either brother or sister, as the younger brother to your elder sister, let us just say this as a prime example. As a child your parents would have your bedroom facing the back garden so that you would not hear the main road traffic as this would lead your parents to sleepiness nights. You are an infant at this moment with a double bedroom, which is highly unfair on your elder sister. You the infant was 3 years old currently, now time for change as your now 9 years old your sister is 13 years old; she wants her space with her accessories of which women like to have make up, mirrors all the elegance to a young princess would acquire. This new change to your adaptation now your bedroom has changed to front house, main road noise and streetlights may take some time getting used to, causing you sleepiness night and a distress.

Going from renting to buying a new property relating anxiety and depression through change of social differences and departure of expenses!

You and your partner have had a stable working-class relationship for some years but have been holding back finances until the time was right to buy a property, of course private renting, has its expenses to pay rent and general household bills!

It has taken years to save for a mortgage deposit and trust being amicable and reciprocated with your partner together! The thought of location can cause a lot of stress and worry without deep research, such as the crime rate within the area, without looking the spec of a house can be a frequent problem to a new family buying a new home with problems if they have not checked these specific spec's details. This can be costly, for example if the bathroom for this instance was not plumbed in as you trusted the seller agent. Another prime example is not underlining your concerns of the possibility of trees canopy, is usually as broad in length as the tree roots will be, also checking distance away from the house the tree is, as an Oak tree can cause crack repairs to the brick work or even damage foundations. Is your house in a location to better your life chances as in opportunities? Do you commute to work? Is the public transport close by? Do you have children? Is there a local school within the area and local activities for children within the community?

<u>A change *of athleticism to a more formal constructive position,*</u>

in your prime your Hobbies becoming your profession, i.e., Running, footballer, bodybuilder you have had to retire due to age and deterioration to your skeletal and muscular system, this has a massive strain on your body slowing heart rate effectively which can play a big part to a mental break down, causing the brain and body anxiety going into panic, long term this can cause you depression as you will not be able to do the things your body was capable of doing before. For when your body breaks down you should never just rely on your physical attributes and find something more therapeutic and simpler for your mind, body, and soul to adjust, such as artwork, reading, furthering your academics to gain cognitive skills. You can gain focus on many things in life which will help you maintain the triumphant feeling of the completion of a medial task. If gaining academics can lead you to a lavish lifestyle, I am quite assured that is the same as winning your home derby football game. I say this as I had experienced the same kind of emotions over time.

The next topic is a little different, but we'll stick with anxiety and depression because most illnesses cause some form of motor neuron disease. state. This leads to muscle weakness and is often accompanied by visible wasting. It occurs when cells stop functioning properly. This is called neurodegeneration. Motor neurons control important muscle activities such as: grasping walking speaking swallowing breathing may eventually become impossible. "As you can see, these symptoms make your daily work unusual compared to the majority! It is a shame to say that it tends to push you into physical labor despite the intense pain it can inflict. have a family history of a related disorder called motor neuron disease or frontotemporal dementia. This is called familial motor neuron disease. In most of these cases, we found that the defective gene contributed significantly to the development of the disease. There is no single test for diagnosing motor neuron disease, and the diagnosis is based on the opinion of a brain and nervous system specialist (neurologist). Diagnosis of motor neuron disease is usually obvious to an experienced neurologist, but

specialist testing may be required to rule out other diseases with similar features. Read more about the causes of motor neuron disease and the diagnosis of motor neuron disease. Symptom Progression Symptoms of motor neuron disease usually start on one side of the body and gradually worsen over weeks to months. Common early symptoms include Weakness in the grip that can make it difficult to lift or hold objects Weakness in the shoulders (dysarthria) that makes it difficult to lift the arm The condition is usually painless. As the damage progresses, symptoms spread to other parts of the body and the condition becomes more debilitating. Finally, people with motor neuron disease can become immobile. Communication, swallowing, and breathing can also be very difficult. In up to 15% of cases, motor neuron disease is associated with a form of dementia that affects personality and behaviour. This is called frontotemporal dementia and is often an early feature with motor neuron disease. Affected people may not realize that their personalities and behaviours are different. Who is affected

by Motor Neuron Disease? is Motor Neuron Disease

<u>Living purely of the ascetics of life!</u>

The simplicity throughout life, living of the highs and lows alone, a chemical imbalance that has serious effects on the motor neurone we have within our brain. Are such substances as, Alcohol, Narcotics. Living with a partner whose suffering from these will have further altercations with your own (positive empathy) of the constant worry, as we know living amongst these suffering come with a fatal consequence such as fatigue, slurred speech, becoming forgetful, emotionless, the making of irrational decisions, making the cost of living hardly bearable. As much as you love your partner it's soul destroying. You cannot commit to supporting these people but only offer advice or point in the right direction. They must want to change themselves and get the help they deserve. Our empathy and compassion come within us all, we all tend to want to help guide and support others, as human citizens our thinking mechanism is to reach out to those who struggle.

I have been and witnessed many single parents who have had a broken-down relationship and one blaming the other through violence of substances such as alcohol and narcotics. Both of which still drink or take narcotics excessively, they are both contradicting others to let them assume they have changed. The story is if you dance with the devil, you get burnt. So many court hearings I have attended from
Hertfordshire constabulary to Colchester Magistrates Court, both courts having non-Molestation orders, witnessing children, father and mother involved. Usual consequences father was verbal or domestic violence. Both with alcoholism and narcotics abuse. Not all but many mothers will end up grasping onto the children regardless as that seems to sit within a family court scenario. The question of simplicity? is, live to the ascetics throughout life, why drink away tomorrow's happiness. Everyone in the World, have different circumstances we face daily, death, blind, born purely disabled or through a tragedy. These innocent people who suffer should become enough for you to want to change. Minus your irreconcilable mind set, this should become

enough to open your eyes to realize how lucky we are. My daily routine has an impact on how I think, how motivated I am, your circle of people, you accompany yourself with, will help you strive or push you to dwell on your lack of positive actions. I attend church ceremony every single Sunday at 9am of Christian Faith. I am also currently studying at Open University, I like to read, write, and work on artwork. Most things being highly creative, an enthusiast, influencer. You need to find your happy place what motivates you as we are all remarkably similar but different in interests and hobbies.

To make change you need to Polaris what you are now? Then to Polaris of where you want to be. What are your ambitions, interests, hobbies, who is your public icon or public influencer, do you see that within reach, within your current circumstances? If not, you need to change that for the better because everything and anything is possible.

If you have a clear conscience.

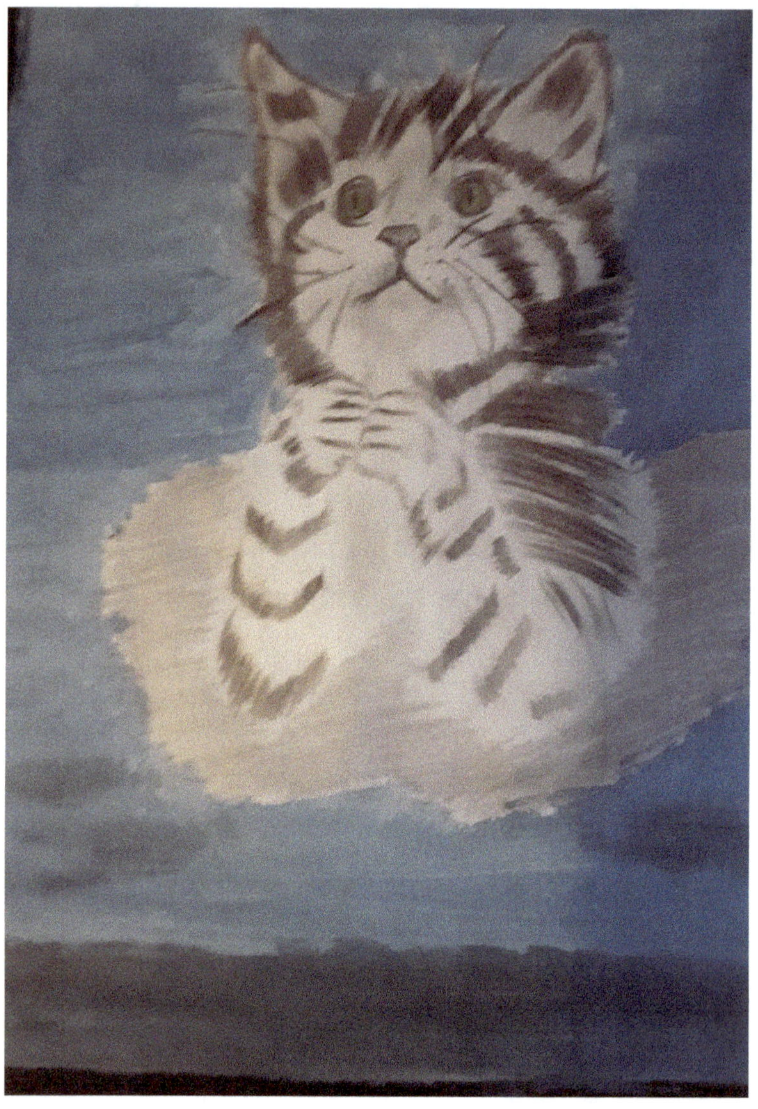

More Impressionist creative artwork via ProcsArt.
Phoenix The CAT.

Interior sacrificial for self-development!

We have gone through half of what can deceive our minds and determine our thoughts, Mental health and being aware of it is particularly important to us all. We need to understand our structure as being apparent, what do you want from out of life? Your aspirations, your goals, and your hobbies. Look at the impacts these will have on your day-to-day living basis? What social circles do they come with? For myself it's too many people, it is too many problems. Family is absolutely everything and supporting them with my compassion, but as a writer and mature student I like to adhere to social media a fair bit, rather than joining social circles from the outside wildlife. I do not drink or take narcotics, so the outside world of the metropolitan lunatic asylum is not for me. Anyhow I have a couple of friends one living in Kent, UK, who works in criminal law, a friend who lives in Cambridge which works in estate Agents, buying and selling property, I've met a nice chap who currently resides in Wales also, who has 2 degrees and looking to do another. He looks after horses as his job preference, a horse whisperer. What I am influencing here is to keep those close to you who inspire you to do well and sacrifice all the people that block your vision. My hobbies are reading, writing, artwork and choir singing. I am a mature student at university, studying arts and humanities. I'm currently a Central Committee Representee for Social Science & Arts Faculty. Every Sunday I am surrounded by positivity within my church community and part of the welcome team/senior side person. I have a passion for the criminal justice system, so I attend Colchester Magistrates Court, this gives me my sanity and most importantly my absolute pleasure and passion to keep writing. When I tend to write with no teleological thoughtful process or logical sense, I literally just like to exfoliate my expression. Creative writing does not come from deep within thought. It simply comes from years of practice. Also, to build aspirations away from anxiety and depression always remembering the "Difficulties in your life do not come to destroy you, they come to help you find your potential to succeed'! Plan, make a vision, make aspirations, set goals and practice methodically! Always remember life is not easy! But its damn sure is how much you want it, to go out there and achieve your dreams. I have been shipwrecked twice or more in my lifetime. Shipwrecked meaning my dreams, aspirations broken down by past relationships, and marriage. Losing a house, clothes, children, cars. It is fine we learn from it. Sometimes failing at a field that is close to your dream it's okay to fail those dreams. Now this is when we build character courage and strength to work on your newly formed character. We as human beings can learn new skills, our intelligence, our mind is as though it is fluorescent, we can make these mistakes then flourish in another field. It is important to find hobbies and interests. Like if you are going for a job position and they say NO never, forget it. It can also mean N.O. Next one, next opportunity.

Keep faith, have no emotions, stay humble, stress and worry are a killer disease if we sit and dwell. 'Think' everything we grew up with within tuition, reading, writing, creativity, mathematics, science, P.E, Technology etc.. The list goes on, take a step back look at your surroundings and prioritize your possibilities regards to your circumstances, it may well be you need to make sacrifices from the company you keep, do not let those be the people that get in your way of an opportunity. Even as we get older, we get into relationships, have children, with a possibility of your child becoming a juvenile, their actions or other actions may bring your mental health to despair. Also remembering we are all carrying burdens upon our shoulders, but when a burden comes Apon the arisen make priorities to build on your aspirations! Never look back at yesterday as tomorrow is anew. Yesterday is in the past, yesterday's failure at life whatever that may be? will not necessarily be tomorrow's success.

Even if someway or somehow you had to make sacrifices to make tomorrow through on your own because of friends, relationship, relatives from your past days made you disorientated! It's intolerable to keep them along with you to reap those rewards by your own accordance. #MakeThatChange today! Do not regret tomorrow. As I narrate my empathy for Mental Health, I cannot help but to acknowledge it is ok not to be ok, as we are our inspiration of becoming apparent with how our mind operates.

Right now I am very fatigued, tiredness, In the UK 12TH August 2022 weathering forecast as hot as the Caribbean the hottest summer to date with a water draught across the Country, I cannot commit to comprehend how elusive and inspirational my thoughts have outlined so much reality context of which I am hoping will help escape the minds and thoughts such as yourself of how and what you might like to change to better yourself as a person or even as a professional. It comes as a sentimental gift from the living of Soley of the ascetics from life, 'the highs and lows. Whatever you dream or passion maybe? Do it with your full potential and do it with pride.

Toxic **Shock Syndrome** Toxic **Shock Syndrome** (TSS) is a rare but life-threatening condition caused by bacteria **entering** the body and releasing harmful toxins. **Often** associated with tampon use in young women, but can affect **people** of **all ages,** including men and children. **Failure to do so** can be **fatal. However, with early diagnosis** and **treatment,** most people **recover completely.** Symptoms of **Toxic Shock Syndrome Symptoms of Toxic Shock Syndrome** (TSS) **begin** suddenly and **worsen**

rapidly. high temperature flu-like **symptoms (headache, chills, fatigue, malaise, body aches,** sore **throat, cough, etc.) nausea** and **vomiting diarrhoea** widespread sunburn-like rash bright red **lips Tongue and Whites of Eyes Dizziness** or **Fainting Difficulty Breathing Confusion Skin that has** bacteria **in** it may **be sore but may** not **appear.**

Seeking Medical Advice Toxic **Shock Syndrome** (TSS) is a medical emergency.

These symptoms **may** be due to **other conditions, but it is** important to contact your GP, local **emergency services** or NHS 111 as soon as possible if these **symptoms are combined. TSS is** very **unlikely,** but these symptoms should not be ignored. **If your symptoms are severe or worsen rapidly, go** to **the** nearest **emergency room** or call 999 **to get** an ambulance **right away.** If **you are** wearing a tampon, remove it **immediately. Also, let** your doctor **know** if you've **used** a tampon, had a **recent** burn or skin injury, or have a skin infection such as a boil. **If doctors suspect her of** TSS, **hospitalize** immediately. **Toxic Shock Syndrome** Treatment If you have **Toxic Shock**

Syndrome (TSS), **you** may need to be **hospitalized and** treated in an intensive care unit. Treatment **of** TSS may **include: Antibiotics** to **Treat Infections In** some cases, purified antibodies taken **from** donated **blood are** given to help **the** body fight **infections. Dehydration** and organ damage **Medications** to control blood pressure **Dialysis** if kidneys **fail In** severe cases, surgery may be needed to remove dead tissue. **In rare cases,** it may be necessary to amputate the affected **area.** Most people **recover** within a few days, but it may take weeks before **they can** leave **the** hospital.

Causes of **poisonous surprise** syndrome Toxic **surprise** syndrome (TSS) is **because of both** staphylococcus or streptococcus **micro organism**. These **micro organism commonly stay at the pores and skin** and **withinside the nostril** or mouth **with out inflicting** harm, **however in the event that they** get deeper into the **frame they could launch pollutants** that **harm** tissue and **forestall** organs working. These **matters** can **boom** your **threat of having** TSS: **the use of** tampons – **mainly in case you depart** them in for longer than **advocated otherwise you** use "super-absorbent" tampons **the use of woman** barrier contraceptives, **which includes** a contraceptive diaphragm or cap a **trouble together along with your pores and skin**, **which includes** a cut, burn, boil, insect **chunk** or a wound after **surgical operation** childbirth **the use of** nasal packing to **deal with** a nosebleed having a staphylococcal **contamination** or streptococcal **contamination**, **which includes** a throat **contamination**, impetigo or cellulitis TSS **isn't always unfold** from **character** to **character**. You do **now no longer increase** immunity to it **as soon as** you've had it, **so that you** can get it **greater** than **as soon as**. Preventing **poisonous surprise** syndrome The following **matters** can **lessen** your **threat** of **poisonous surprise** syndrome (TSS): **deal with** wounds and burns **speedy** and get **scientific recommendation in case you observe symptoms and symptoms** of an **contamination**, **which includes** swelling, redness and **growing ache** Always use a tampon with **the bottom** absorbency **appropriate to your duration change among** tampons and a sanitary towel or panty liner **at some point of** your **duration** wash your **arms earlier than** and after **placing** a tampon **extrade** tampons regularly – as

frequently as directed **at the** pack (**generally at the least each four to eight** hours) Never have **multiple** tampon **on your** vagina at a time When **the use of** a tampon at night, insert a **sparkling** tampon **earlier than** going to **mattress** and **dispose of** it **whilst you awaken dispose of** a tampon **on the give up** of your **duration whilst the use of woman** barrier **birth control**, **comply with** the manufacturer's **commands approximately** how **lengthy you could depart** it in It's an **progressive concept** to **keep away from the use of** tampons or **woman** barrier **birth control when you have** had TSS **earlier than**.

- With our Mental Health and wellbeing in mind, it's incredibly important to stay focused, some formality of exercise, watching what we eat, drinking plenty of fluids such as water, In the way that we act and the way we treat each other simplifies how we treat ourselves. The motto of life and your stability with your Mental health and wellbeing is what you put in (Fuel assumptions of food & drink) is what you get out, start to polarize a better way of living. If you make better eating habits &

drinking habits, you will start to treat people better, you also feel more confident in how you feel about yourself, more motivation, more compassion, and empathy to care and help one another when times of struggle. We all need mental health, if you have no mental health awareness or any kind of acknowledgment and how will you understand when you are having a chemical imbalance or when life is running smoothly. We ae certainly not all masters of our own minds, there are times in our lives that not all of us have received the same life sentence, some of us may lost grandparents, aunts, uncles, sister, brother, wife, or husband, some of us may had many tragic such as car crashes, sport injuries, falling of a push bike, raped, stabbed etc.. I will not keep on, but it is how we counter act the defects that can occur in our life that can physically damage us for life, if we dwell too much on yesterday's incident, you're going to make Tomorrow just as worse, road to recovery why dwell on yesterday when tomorrow is anew. Listening to the fact that alcohol and narcotics is not a substitute to take away the pain, it may or may well not, the next day the pain shall hit you a lot worse and more than likely have an added hangover. Time and forbearance is the only cure, I thrive of compassion, there are 7.9 billion people within the entire world, have a look around there is so much trauma throughout societies in other Countries a lot worse of then you, water draught, food shortages, fires, floods, these second world countries watching their baby brother starve to death at the side of the road awaiting for a food delivery, many dying at the side of the road awaiting a delivery of water, dying of thirst. In Nigeria children being part of one the world's biggest human traffic invention, Children in Africa get bribed into sex to get granted their tuition. This information provided may not be 1 million percent wholly correct, but I can assure you this is what we are seeing daily in the media.

Living through life of resentment?

Forgive yourself for what you allowed and for the things you had no control over. Letting go of resentment does not diminish what they did to you. In fact, letting go allows you to take your power back- Ash Alves, Resentment is nasty. What makes it so ugly is that is has a tendency to turn you into an otherwise kind and reasonable person, into someone who is so angry at their own life situation that it is nearly impossible to recover.

Bitterness and resentment make it hard even for the people who love you to be around you- Martha Body felt.

"Resentment is a very hard thing to live with. Many people can hide behind a lie, some people lie so much they believe their lies are telling the truth. Resentment comes as a form of jealousy, hurt and anger towards another being. The person who resents you may be jealous of what you're trying to accomplish. Many a woman or a man will suffice resentment throughout work, relationships, hobbies, or interests because the other is doing what you want to accomplish.

Always remember to not become narcissistic with feeling resentment is a one-sided thing. Hurt and anger are the majority of the time two sides to the situation 9 times out of 10. Life is about building one another, not bringing each other's values down."

(Some people I wish I could understand their actions. Their hurt, their anger. But then there is some people you just have to shut the door and never look back). Hatred is a complex, diverse feeling that has been portrayed as a combination of frustration, repugnance, outrage, and dread. Different clinicians think of it as a state of mind or as an optional inclination (includ…

Hatred considers inadequately you and adds to the cynicism of the workplace, an endless loop that can contribute much more to your harshness.

Feelings of hatred resemble weeds which are well established and develop effectively, they ruin connections, and they make us unpleasant and detached.

Self-growth and Hatred feelings coming from resentment can likewise turn into a reason for not assuming command over our own lives and we can utilize our feelings of disdain to jab the finger of fault at others for why we are not carrying on with the daily routine we need to experience. Resentment is most difficult when it is felt toward an individual, you are near, like a parent, old friend, or life partner. If you do not beat sensations of feebleness, you could foster a negative, threatening disposition.

Hatred is extreme, particularly when you've been wounded by somebody profoundly. We as a whole battle with disdain eventually in our lives. However, when we clutch outrage and disdain, it just goals us to experience more. What you may not understand is that disdain can significantly affect your physical and psychological wellness. Holding hard feelings makes us convey pessimistic, tense energy in our science.

"At the point when we clutch hard feelings and hatred, it resembles drinking poison and anticipating that the other individual should become ill. "You should focus on your degrees of hatred. Resulting in it unrestrained can harm you in additional ways than you know. The following are four diverse ways disdain influences your wellbeing.

It places you in survival mode.

An unbelievable actual weight too is being harmed and frustrated. At the point when you're persistently furious and clutch disdain, it can place you into survival mode. This can cause momentous changes in your circulatory strain, pulse, and resistant reaction. At the point when these things happen, it can expand the gamble of gloom, diabetes, coronary illness, and other conditions. Pardoning can turn this around, as absolution further develops feelings of anxiety and prompts better wellbeing generally speaking.

It causes mental harm.

At the point when we convey disdain and gloomy feelings like sharpness and outrage, it can cause mental harm. At the point when we harp on these sentiments, it can start to annihilate our mentality and check others out. You will start to check out at everything through a negative focal point. Hatred likewise keeps us intellectually trapped before, which keeps us from pushing ahead. This can hinder your capacity to see the valuable open doors before you. You might try and start to see yourself in a negative light. This isn't just undesirable yet additionally damaging.

It annihilates connections.

Hatred can obliterate your character, which will influence your companionships and associations with friends and family. You start to turn into nobody's desired individual to invest energy in, and you wind up feeling more alone.

: Instructions to Utilize the Most Significant Piece of Your Mind Under Any Sort of Pressure," says that furious and angry individuals cause problems, especially in close connections, in any event, when they are not doing anything wrong.

This is on the grounds that their bodies and looks commonly express dissatisfaction and aggression beyond their mindfulness. "Being around furious and angry individuals makes us angry, in any event, when they say nothing hostile, "While you're clinging to disdain, individuals around you notice, regardless of whether you understand it.

It makes us have more pessimistic feelings.

On the off chance that you're clutching outrage and hatred, you'll wind up encountering many gloomy feelings. The significance of relinquishing outrage on account of the harm it causes to our wellbeing. "Individuals who are furious a ton will quite often have other persistent gloomy feelings too,". "Relinquishing hatred can assist with upgrading your wellbeing without you in any event, taking note. The most effective way to push ahead from hatred is to track down evident bliss. Quite possibly of everything thing you can manage to break liberated from the chains of hatred is to pardon. It is finished for our own bliss and development. At the point when we clutch our aggravation, it truly hurts more the individual clutching it than any other person. At the point when we pardon, we can continue on without wanting to look for vengeance or disdain for the individual that incurred our aggravation.

At the point when we decide to pardon, that doesn't imply that we are legitimizing the hurtful way of behaving. It likewise doesn't imply that we will keep on connecting with the individual that hurt us similarly. Notwithstanding, it implies that we are liberating ourselves from a gigantic weight that influences our wellbeing and our perspective.

At the point when we decide not to pardon an individual who hurt us or violated us, we start to take on so many gloomy feelings that can harm us genuinely, intellectually, and inwardly. Investigations have discovered that absolution has enormous medical advantages. Research likewise brings up that this can increase with age. "Pardoning" is a decision, "You are deciding to offer sympathy and compassion to the individual who violated you." If you dislike somebody, you should start to do whatever it may take to change your demeanour so your physical and psychological well-being can get to the next level.

You can start to do this through the demonstration of reflection. Glance back at the occasions that have occurred in your life that make you battle with outrage and disdain. Contemplate the manners in which you have felt and responded to those circumstances. Ask yourself what these circumstances mean for you now.

Additionally, find opportunity to feel for the individual you are irate with or disdaining. If you have any desire to pardon and start the mending system, it very well might be an ideal opportunity to converse with that individual. You should not stroll into these circumstances with any assumptions. Keep in mind, a conciliatory sentiment may not come from that individual. Getting an expression of remorse ought not be the objective.

Your mending ought to. At the point when you don't come into circumstances with assumptions, you won't ever be frustrated.

At the point when you choose to pardon, you are transforming your sentiments into activities. Pardoning is an interaction that requires some investment. It's not something you accomplish for the individual who hurt you, however for you. It's likewise critical that you require the investment to excuse yourself. Individuals frequently fail to remember that the demonstration of pardoning likewise incorporates the absolution of self. Any aggravation you felt because of somebody's activities isn't an impression of your value.

Can Money buy happiness?

A life of aloofness, or a life of solidarity recognition?
The difference to compare both within evidence.
To stand proud and aloof drained physically and mentally detached a figure, to a life that is full of compromised middle-class spectators being fed

from a silver spoon to bring your solitude of full-fill ness amid amongst a Hurd of sheep.

Isn't it ironic what money can buy? Money can buy you simply an estranged upgrade within a prison cell. Money can buy pride, money can buy triumph, money can buy friends.
Doing something volunteering, the time, the perseverance, the observance, and the passion shall slide others eagle eyes and deceit you. But nevertheless, a volunteering job comes with compassion and a feel-good factor of supporting the community. Have a think of what money cannot buy, pride, passion, integrity, compassion and a full-fillness and empathy on striving within the community. To build an amicable and reciprocated Relationship you need to be able to relate, you have the same quantity's, qualities of passion making monies or serving the community through pure pride, passion, integrity, compassion, the kind-hearted volunteering perspective perhaps? You will then probably find a more suitable coalition between the two recipients from within the pair of etiquette

occupants, to form its true allegiance within the volunteering sector.

Money can be fulfilling, it can buy you many things, but money can also become lavishly greed over what we deem as necessarily. Money can also become as resentful for others also who work all the voluntary hours under the sun, for some claim of recognition. You need to claim what works best for your ability, your Mental Health & well-being. Do not try to bite off more than you can chew, accept what is or what can become achievable within your limits, try not to proclaim to much energy into several opportunity's that within itself can drive your energy to fatigue and your mentality will start to fall. Compensating too much for recognition. It is time to focus on what is or what could become, you can become an acceptance if you strive through one field with excellence. Trying to plough to many fields will become exacerbated and common faultless.

It’s time to take a self-reflection of your aspirations, goals, mindset, your capabilities, and your wellbeing. With your current circumstances, ie caring for parents, children, what hobbies or interests you may or may not have put all that in your time frame perspective then decide what is now insight of aspirations and achievements.

With Blemishing & flourishing scripture you'll discover a mentality to what you could suffice, Health & vitality is more admirable a solitude which we can best perform self-development, but too much loneliness could deplete our mentality into depression, so I would care to some apparent social interaction. There is a fine line of self-development and caring for your mental wellbeing. The thought of lonesome dark nights a drift, the summer's day over the country park escalating boredom the event to be accompanied by other adults with same interests and hobbies sometimes feels more appropriate. #

Words of wisdom!, if you accept bible scripture or not? I spent time observing characters and life struggles to influence you to a better focused lifestyle, with fundamentals to actions and plans to help with a fluent productive mindset.

The Serenity Prayer God grant me the serenity to[1] accept the things I cannot change; Courage to change the things I can; And wisdom to know the difference. Living one day at a time; Enjoying one moment at a time; Accepting hardships as the pathway to peace; Taking, as He did, this sinful world as it is, not as I would have it; Trusting that He will make all things right If I surrender to His Will; So that I may be reasonably happy in this life and supremely happy with Him Forever and ever in the next.

James 3:13
13 Who is wise and understanding among you? Let them show it by their good life, by deeds done in the humility that comes from wisdom.

Proverbs 4:7
7 The beginning of wisdom is this: Get wisdom. Though it cost all you have, get understanding.

Proverbs 11:2

---

[1] Mind Matters/Writer/Author/J.Johnson

2 When pride comes, then comes disgrace, but with humility comes wisdom.

Proverbs 16:16

16 How much better to get wisdom than gold, to get insight rather than silver!

Proverbs 17:28

28 Even fools are thought wise if they keep silent, and discerning if they hold their tongues.

Proverbs 19:8

8 The one who gets wisdom loves life; the one who cherishes understanding will soon prosper.

Proverbs 13:10

10 Where there is strife, there is pride, but wisdom is found in those who take advice.

Psalms 37:30

30 The mouths of the righteous utter wisdom, and their tongues speak what is just.

Ephesians 5:15-16

15 Be very careful, then, how you live—not as unwise but as wise,

16 making the most of every opportunity, because the days are evil.

Beating anxiety, depression, the hurt the pain and anger.
Fuelling the mind through vitality, looking after your fuel consumption, being careful of what we eat and drink, making sure we are nourished to utilize our fully functioning body and mind. Drinking on average 2 litre of water a day. I like to use cod liver oils for my synovial joints to keep them lubricated. Fish foods have many beneficial effects for our body to function such as our joints and our mind.

How many calories should the average person intake daily? The number of calories the body consumes in a day is different for every person. You may notice on the nutritional labels of the foods you buy that the "percent daily values" are based on a 2,000-calorie diet -- 2,000 calories are a rough average of what people eat in a day. But your body might need more or less than 2,000. The eat well plate below gives you an idea of the ideas of what percentage your plate should be covered by Carbohydrates, Protein, Fats, not forgetting your 5 a day.

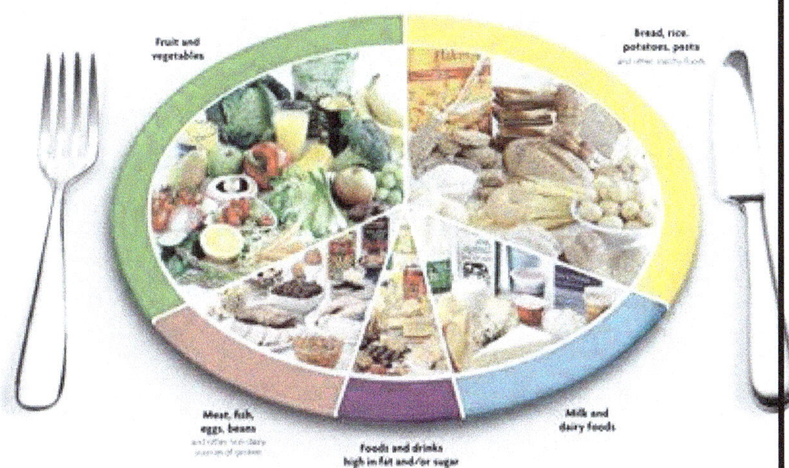

With some of my useful tools, information ideas I am hoping you can make an action plan which works best for you, supporting your mental Health & Wellbeing, chosen your hobbies, interests what circle of people do you want and need to get your aspirations out of life. I really hope you have now thought about your lifestyle, is it appropriate or inappropriate, what could you do better? What could be a prodigious invention to help me flourish. You want to use some of the ideas to help you progress as a person. To gain your vitality, Your strengths within your Mental Health & Well-being. Ideas how to keep the mind active, ideas how to fuel the body and mind. Ideas on how to keep positive thoughts in the mind, choosing your circle of friends. What kind of friends do you want in your boat? And want kind of friends would be best left ashore? You need friends that can only bring to your life and inspire you to do well. As soon as they're not willing to participate with accepting that, then that friendship needs to become annihilated.

Mental **health needs** to **be talked** about more than **ever. Especially** as we **are starting** to **realize** the impact Covid 19 has had on **us and** all the **children who** have missed so much **in recent years such as** education and socializing with friends. Here **are** some ways families can support each **other.**

* **Deep breathing is very helpful in relaxing** and **calming** the **body.**

* **Being** active helps **give your** brain **a boost** as the chemicals released help **create a** positive **mood. Find** an activity **that works for** you and your child.

* **"Worry Box"** helps **to** get rid of **troubles.** You can support your child by helping **with decorating** and **taking care of** their worries.

***Front facing glasses are good for children. Fill the** jar with lots of happy **thoughts, messages, ideas,** and **statements. Talk** about what makes you happy.

***Socializing** and spending time **just by reading, cuddling in front of the** TV, going for a **walk,** or just being **together** can **improve a child's mood and keep them** a consistent and positive presence.

Mental Health Awareness Listen **to** some **people.** They come into your life to **take advantage of you.** They **don't** come to bring **something into** your **life. they will rob** you. They **don't** see you as a **person. They** see you as an **opportunity.** They love you for what they can take from **you. They** are not loyal to **you. They should benefit from what** they **get** from **you. So,** no matter how many times you **show** up for **them,** they never **show up. How real.** Stop breaking your **back** for people **who** clearly **don't** get **what's yours. I** live by **it,** but you **don't** have to live by it. **Otherwise, the** relationship **must** be **destroyed. Use is prohibited. So,** stop taking punches from people who **won't** take **punches** from **you.** Stop **getting** people **on** your boat **who won't roll** with you. Stop being there for **those who have disappeared** from you. I hate to say **this,** but **the**

reality is that if they **don't support** you, they **don't matter** in your life. **Straight.** Just because someone is in your life **doesn't** mean they want **to make the most** of your life. **Let** me ask you **a question. Would it still be there if it weren't for your talent?** If **you weren't depressed in life,** would they be **depressed** for you? **Most of all, what** you have to offer is friendship. **are** they still **there**

I know you want their support, but **you are** not **getting** it. But understand **that** you **do not** need their support. I know it sucks when you find **that** the **person** you love the **most is** the **person who supports** you the least. **Well,** I know **it's boring** to **know who I've** done the least **for.** But **they should** not **lack support. For those just embracing talent, it should not be a** lack of **relief. I** want to use **that much. Bypass** people who **not only want to drink from your cup, but also** want to pour into your cup. **Meet** people who want to **improve** your life, not **people** who **just** want to **improve their life. Don't keep runaways** in your life **who** expect everything from you but give **you nothing. You don't understand that** well, **who is** there to support you? There is a **world** full of people **who are rooting for you.** So **do not** let **people who do not** support you stop you from **watching this. Eliminate** these people from your **life and it** will. They try to paint you **a wrong picture of life! when** they **have wronged you.** I want you to understand that I **will** never forget, **and I will** never feel guilty. **Cutting** someone off when handed scissors. **as i** always **say.** It all starts with you; **it is time for rehab. Go** there and get it. Anyone else **able** to **comment? Like** my life as a **child.** I struggled **all through** school, **but** when I **finished school,** I went into **construction and all sports. It is** the sucker **that feels the pain. Today,** everyone **suffers from pain** in some **form** or **another.** And let me tell you **they** help.

But **there is also extraordinarily little** help we can get. **It is exceedingly difficult** to **obtain.** But **even here we must fight. But you need** to want it and accept the help you can **get. You need to scream** for help before **it is** too late.

Useful contacts

Mind's services

- Mind's helplines provide information and support by phone and email.
- Local Minds offer face-to-face services across England and Wales. These services include talking therapies, peer support and advocacy.
- Side by Side is our supportive online community for anyone experiencing a mental health problem.

Other organisations
Anxiety UK

Advice and support for people living with anxiety
Beat

British Association for Counselling and Psychotherapy (BACP) bacp.co.uk
Professional body for talking therapy and counselling. Provides information and a list of accredited therapists.

Campaign Against Living Miserably (CALM)

Provides listening services, information, and support for anyone who needs to talk, including a web chat.

Carers UK
0808 808 7777
029 2081 1370 (Carers Wales)

Advice and support for anyone who provides care.

Information and support for people living with a disability.

FRANK

Confidential advice and information about drugs, their effects and the law.

Information and support for people affected by mental health problems in Wales.

Hearing Voices Network hearing-voices.org
Information and support for people who hear voices or have other unshared perceptions, including local support groups.

Mental health service run by and for LGBTQ+ people.

National Institute for Health and Care Excellence (NICE) nice.org.uk
Produces guidelines on best practice in healthcare.

Information about health problems and treatments, including details of local NHS services in England.

No Panic

Provides a helpline, step-by-step programmes, and support for people with anxiety disorders.

Papyrus HOPELINEUK

Freepost SAMARITANS
LETTERS
samaritans.org

Samaritans are open 24/7 for anyone who needs to talk. You can visit some Samaritans branches in person. Samaritans also have a Welsh Language Line on 0808 164 0123 (7pm–11pm every day).

Offers emotional support and information for anyone affected by mental health problems.

t
Mental health charity that supports students.

Time to Change time-to-change.org.uk (England) timetochangewales.org.uk (Wales)
National campaign to end stigma and discrimination against people with mental health problems in England and Wales. The campaign for England ended in 2021, but its resources are still available -point.co.uk

Health and social care services in England for people with a learning disability. Also supports people with mental health problems, drug and alcohol abuse or unemployment.

YoungMinds
0808 802 5544 (Parents Helpline)
85258 (Crisis Messenger for young people – text the letters YM) youngminds.org.uk
Committed to improving the mental health of babies, children and young people, including support for parents and carers.

If you just need to talk, any time of day or night

Free listening services

These services offer confidential support from trained volunteers. You can talk about anything that's troubling no matter how difficult:

- Call 116 123 to talk to Samaritans, or email: jo@samaritans.org for a reply within 24
- hours
- Text "SHOUT" to 85258 to contact the
- Shout Crisis Text Line, or text "YM" if you're
- under 19

If you're under 19, you can also call 0800 1111 to talk to Childline. The number will not appear on your

phone bill.

Make sure you plan to try and better your Mental Health & Well-being, remember plenty of sleep, stay hydrated not intoxicated, exercise minimal 2hours per week and eat well remembering your 5 a day.

The eat-well plate gives you some ides what your plate should consist of, remembering average calories intake is roughly 2500 on the average person.

You can find us on___________-------

'Facebook' Proclamtion Johnson'
'Instagram' j.johnson.39
'YouTube' Proclamation news and Gatherence

Welcome to leave us some constructive criticism.
I believe no book is finished without feedback as I wan
reach out to others who are or who have suffered Ment
Health Illness in the past.

Welcome to share your experience's
This is currently my first authored book, we are
aiming to produce a second running on book
called 'nursing mind matters 2.
within the new year of 2023, I have been a sufferer of
Mental Health illness myself. But it is how
we maintain it that's all that matters.
' It is ok not to be okay',
just make sure you call for help.

www.ingramcontent.com/pod-product-compliance
Lightning Source LLC
Chambersburg PA
CBHW071329310526
45789CB00017B/2119

* 9 7 8 1 4 7 1 0 6 8 5 2 2 *